THE MEDITERRANEAN DIET COOKBOOK MEAT RECIPES

Quick, Easy and Tasty Recipes to feel full of energy, stay healthy keeping your weight under control

Melanie Castelli

Copyright © 2021 by Melanie Castelli

All right reserved. No part of this publication may be reproduced in any form without permission in writing form the publisher, except for brief quotations used for publishable articles or reviews.

Legal Disclaimer

The information contained in this book and its contents is not designed to replace any form of medical or professional advice; and is not meant to replace the need for independent medical, financial, legal, or other professional advice or service that may require. The content and information in this book have been provided for educational and entertainment purposes only.

The content and information contained in this book have been compiled from sources deemed reliable, and they are accurate to the best of the Author's knowledge, information and belief.

However, the Author cannot guarantee its accuracy and validity and therefore cannot be held liable for any errors and/or omissions.

Further, changes are periodically made to this book as needed. Where appropriate and/or necessary, you must consult a professional (including but not limited to your doctor, attorney, financial advisor, or other such professional) before using any of the suggested remedies, techniques, and/or information in this book.

Upon using this book's contents and information, you agree to hold harmless the Author from any damaged, costs and expenses, including any legal fees potentially resulting from the application of any of the information in this book. This disclaimer applies to any loss, damages, or injury caused by the use and application of this book's content, whether directly and indirectly, whether for breach of contract, tort, negligence, personal injury, criminal intent, or under any other circumstances.

You agree to accept all risks of using the information presented in this book. You agree that by continuing to read this book, where appropriate and/or necessary, you shall consult a professional (including but not limited to your doctor, attorney, financial advisor, or other such professional) before remedies, techniques, and/or information in this book.

TABLE OF CONTENTS

MAIN RECIPES: MEAT 8
Grilled Chicken Breasts 8
Buttery Garlic Chicken 10
Creamy Chicken-Spinach Skillet 12
Slow Cooker Mediterranean Beef Roast 14
Slow Cooker Mediterranean Beef with Artichokes 16
Slow Cooker Meatloaf 18
Slow Cooker Mediterranean Beef Hoagies 20
Beef & Bulgur Meatballs 23
Tasty Beef and Broccoli 25
Soy Sauce Beef Roast 26
Mediterranean Grilled Pork Chops 28
Simple Pork Stir Fry 30
Pork and Lentil Soup 32
Simple Braised Pork 34
Pork and Chickpea Stew 37
Pork and Greens Salad 39
Pork Strips and Rice 40
Slow Cooked Mediterranean Pork 42
Pork and Bean Stew 44

The Mediterranean Diet Cookbook: Meat Recipes

Pork with Couscous 46

Grilled Steak, Mushroom, and Onion Kebabs 48

Turkey Meatballs 50

Chicken Marsala 52

Cauliflower Steaks with Eggplant Relish 54

Lemon Caper Chicken 56

Herb Roasted Chicken 58

Mediterranean bowl 60

Tasty Lamb Leg 62

Kale Sprouts & Lamb 64

Grilled Harissa Chicken 65

Italian Chicken Meatballs 67

Classic Chicken Cooking with Tomatoes & Tapenade 70

Turkish Turkey Mini Meatloaves 72

Charred Chicken Souvlaki Skewers 74

Mediterranean Lamb Chops 76

Mushroom and Beef Risotto 78

Oven Roasted Garlic Chicken Thigh 80

Balearic Beef Brisket Bowl 82

Grilled Grapes & Chicken Chunks 84

Mediterranean Beef Skewers 86

Cumin Lamb Mix 88

Beef & Potatoes 89

Pork and Chestnuts Mix 90

Rosemary Pork Chops 91

The Mediterranean Diet Cookbook: Meat Recipes

Tender Lamb 92

Worcestershire Pork Chops 94

Greek Pork 95

Pork with Green Beans & Potatoes 96

Beef and Chili Mix 97

Greek Meatballs 98

Mediterranean Lamb Bowl 99

Lamb Burger 101

Quick Herbed Lamb and Pasta 103

Marinated Lamb Kebabs with Crunchy Yogurt Dressing 105

Garlic Pork Tenderloin and Lemony Orzo 107

Roasted Pork with Apple-Dijon Sauce 108

The Mediterranean Diet Cookbook: Meat Recipes

MAIN RECIPES: MEAT

Grilled Chicken Breasts

Preparation Time: 10 minutes
Cooking Time: 15 minutes
Servings: 2
INGREDIENTS:
- Boneless skinless chicken breast, 4.
- Lemon juice, 3 tbsp.
- Olive oil, 3 tbsp.
- Chopped fresh parsley, 3 tbsp.
- Minced garlic cloves, 3.
- Paprika, 1 tsp.
- Dried oregano, ½ tsp.
- Salt and pepper, to taste.

DIRECTIONS:
1. In a large Ziploc bag, mix well oregano, paprika, garlic, parsley, olive oil, and lemon juice.
2. Pierce chicken with a knife several times and sprinkle with salt and pepper.

3. Add chicken to bag and marinate 20 minutes or up to two days in the fridge.
4. Remove chicken from bag and grill for 5 minutes per side in a 3500 F preheated grill.
5. When cooked, transfer to a plate for 5 minutes before slicing.
6. Serve and enjoy with a side of rice or salad

NUTRITION: Calories: 238, Protein: 24 g, Carbohydrates: 2 g, Fats: 19 g

Buttery Garlic Chicken

Preparation Time: 5 minutes
Cooking Time: 40 minutes

Servings: 2

INGREDIENTS:

- ✓ 2 tablespoons ghee, melted
- ✓ 2 boneless skinless chicken breasts
- ✓ tablespoon dried Italian seasoning
- ✓ 4 tablespoons butter
- ✓ ¼ cup grated Parmesan cheese

DIRECTIONS:

1. Preheat the oven to 375°F. Select a baking dish that fit both chicken breasts and coat it with the ghee.
2. Pat dries the chicken breasts. Season with pink Himalayan salt, pepper, and Italian seasoning. Place the chicken in the baking dish.
3. In a medium skillet over medium heat, melt the butter. Sauté minced garlic, for about 5 minutes.
4. Remove the butter-garlic mixture from the heat, and pour it over the chicken breasts.

5. Roast in the oven for 30 to 35 minutes. Sprinkle some of the Parmesan cheese on top of each chicken breast. Let the chicken rest in the baking dish for 5 minutes.
6. Divide the chicken between two plates, spoon the butter sauce over the chicken, and serve.

NUTRITION: 642 Calories 45g Fat 57g Protein

Creamy Chicken-Spinach Skillet

Preparation Time: 10 minutes

Cooking Time: 17 minutes

Servings: 2

INGREDIENTS:

- ✓ Boneless skinless chicken breast, 1 lb.
- ✓ Medium diced onion, 1.
- ✓ Diced roasted red peppers, 12 oz.
- ✓ Chicken stock, 2 ½ cups.
- ✓ Baby spinach leaves, 2 cups.
- ✓ Cooked pasta, 2 cups.
- ✓ Butter, 2 tbsp.
- ✓ Minced garlic cloves, 4.
- ✓ Cream cheese, 7 oz.
- ✓ Salt and pepper, to taste.

DIRECTIONS:

1. Place a saucepan on medium high heat for 2 minutes. Add butter and melt for a minute, swirling to coat the pan.
2. Add chicken to a pan, season with pepper and salt to taste. Cook chicken on high heat for 3 minutes per side.

3. Lower heat to medium and stir in onions, red peppers, and garlic. Sauté for 5 minutes and deglaze pot with a little bit of stock.
4. Whisk in chicken stock and cream cheese. Cook and mix until thoroughly combined.
5. Stir in spinach and adjust seasoning to taste. Cook for 2 minutes or until spinach is wilted.
6. Serve and enjoy.

NUTRITION: Calories: 484, Protein: 36 g, Carbohydrates: 33 g, Fats: 22 g

Slow Cooker Mediterranean Beef Roast

Preparation Time: 10 minutes

Cooking Time: 10 hours and 10 minutes

Servings: 2

INGREDIENTS:

- ✓ 3 pounds Chuck roast, boneless
- ✓ 2 teaspoons Rosemary
- ✓ ½ cup Tomatoes, sun-dried and chopped
- ✓ 10 cloves Grated garlic
- ✓ ½ cup Beef stock
- ✓ 2 tablespoons Balsamic vinegar
- ✓ ¼ cup Chopped Italian parsley, fresh
- ✓ ¼ cup Chopped olives
- ✓ 1 teaspoon Lemon zest
- ✓ ¼ cup Cheese grits

DIRECTIONS:

- In the slow cooker, put garlic, sun dried tomatoes, and the beef roast. Add beef stock and Rosemary. Close the cooker and slow cook for 10 hours.
- After cooking is over, remove the beef, and shred the meet. Discard the fat. Add back the shredded

meat to the slow cooker and simmer for 10 minutes.
- In a small bowl combine lemon zest, parsley, and olives. Cool the mixture until you are ready to serve. Garnish using the refrigerated mix.
- Serve it over pasta or egg noodles. Top it with cheese grits.

NUTRITION: 314 Calories 19g Fat 1g Carbohydrate 32g Protein 778mg Sodium

Slow Cooker Mediterranean Beef with Artichokes

Preparation Time: 3 hours and 20 minutes

Cooking Time: **7 hours and 8 minutes**

Servings: 2

INGREDIENTS:

- ✓ 2 pounds Beef for stew
- ✓ 14 ounces Artichoke hearts
- ✓ 1 tablespoon Grape seed oil
- ✓ 1 Diced onion
- ✓ 32 ounces Beef broth
- ✓ 4 cloves Garlic, grated
- ✓ 14½ ounces Tinned tomatoes, diced
- ✓ 15 ounces Tomato sauce
- ✓ 1 teaspoon Dried oregano
- ✓ ½ cup Pitted, chopped olives
- ✓ 1 teaspoon Dried parsley
- ✓ 1 teaspoon Dried oregano
- ✓ ½ teaspoon Ground cumin
- ✓ 1 teaspoon Dried basil
- ✓ 1 Bay leaf

- ✓ ½ teaspoon Salt

DIRECTIONS:

1. In a large non-stick skillet pour some oil and bring to medium-high heat. Roast the beef until it turns brown on both the sides. Transfer the beef into a slow cooker.

NUTRITION: 314 Calories 19g Fat 1g Carbohydrate 32g Protein 778mg Sodium

Slow Cooker Meatloaf

Preparation Time: 10 minutes

Cooking Time: 6 hours and 10 minutes

Servings: 2

INGREDIENTS:

- ✓ 2 pounds Ground bison
- ✓ 1 Grated zucchini
- ✓ 2 large Eggs
- ✓ Olive oil cooking spray as required
- ✓ 1 Zucchini, shredded
- ✓ ½ cup Parsley, fresh, finely chopped
- ✓ ½ cup Parmesan cheese, shredded
- ✓ 3 tablespoons Balsamic vinegar
- ✓ 4 Garlic cloves, grated
- ✓ 2 tablespoons Onion minced
- ✓ 1 tablespoon Dried oregano
- ✓ ½ teaspoon Ground black pepper
- ✓ ½ teaspoon Kosher salt
- ✓ For the topping:
- ✓ ¼ cup Shredded Mozzarella cheese
- ✓ ¼ cup Ketchup without sugar

- ✓ ¼ cup Freshly chopped parsley

DIRECTIONS:

1. Stripe line the inside of a six-quart slow cooker with aluminum foil. Spray non-stick cooking oil over it.
2. In a large bowl combine ground bison or extra lean ground sirloin, zucchini, eggs, parsley, balsamic vinegar, garlic, dried oregano, sea or kosher salt, minced dry onion, and ground black pepper.
3. Situate this mixture into the slow cooker and form an oblong shaped loaf. Cover the cooker, set on a low heat and cook for 6 hours. After cooking, open the cooker and spread ketchup all over the meatloaf.
4. Now, place the cheese above the ketchup as a new layer and close the slow cooker. Let the meatloaf sit on these two layers for about 10 minutes or until the cheese starts to melt. Garnish with fresh parsley, and shredded Mozzarella cheese.

NUTRITION: 320 Calories 2g Fat 4g Carbohydrates 26g Protein 681mg Sodium

Slow Cooker Mediterranean Beef Hoagies

Preparation Time: 10 minutes
Cooking Time: 13 hours
Servings: 2

INGREDIENTS:

- ✓ 3 pounds Beef top round roast fatless
- ✓ ½ teaspoon Onion powder
- ✓ ½ teaspoon Black pepper
- ✓ 3 cups Low sodium beef broth
- ✓ 4 teaspoons Salad dressing mix
- ✓ 1 Bay leaf
- ✓ 1 tablespoon Garlic, minced
- ✓ 2 Red bell peppers, thin strips cut
- ✓ 16 ounces Pepperoncino
- ✓ 8 slices Sargento Provolone, thin
- ✓ 2 ounces Gluten-free bread
- ✓ ½ teaspoon salt
- ✓ For seasoning:
- ✓ 1½ tablespoon Onion powder
- ✓ 1½ tablespoon Garlic powder

- ✓ 2 tablespoon Dried parsley
- ✓ 1 tablespoon stevia
- ✓ ½ teaspoon Dried thyme
- ✓ 1 tablespoon Dried oregano
- ✓ 2 tablespoons Black pepper
- ✓ 1 tablespoon Salt
- ✓ 6 Cheese slices

DIRECTIONS:

1. Dry the roast with a paper towel. Combine black pepper, onion powder and salt in a small bowl and rub the mixture over the roast.
2. Place the seasoned roast into a slow cooker.
3. Add broth, salad dressing mix, bay leaf, and garlic to the slow cooker. Combine it gently. Close and set to low cooking for 12 hours. After cooking, remove the bay leaf.
4. Take out the cooked beef and shred the beef meet. Put back the shredded beef and add bell peppers and. Add bell peppers and pepperoncino into the slow cooker.
5. Cover the cooker and low cook for 1 hour. Before serving, top each of the bread with 3 ounces of

the meat mixture. Top it with a cheese slice. The liquid gravy can be used as a dip.

NUTRITION: 442 Calories 11.5g Fat 37g Carbohydrates 49g Protein 735mg Sodium

Beef & Bulgur Meatballs

Preparation Time: 20 minutes

Cooking Time: 28 minutes

Servings: 2

INGREDIENTS:

- ¾ cup uncooked bulgur
- 1-pound ground beef
- ¼ cup shallots, minced
- ¼ cup fresh parsley, minced
- ½ teaspoon ground allspice
- ½ teaspoon ground cumin
- ½ teaspoon ground cinnamon
- ¼ teaspoon red pepper flakes, crushed
- Salt, as required
- 1 tablespoon olive oil

DIRECTIONS:

1. In a large bowl of the cold water, soak the bulgur for about 30 minutes. Drain the bulgur well and then, squeeze with your hands to remove the excess water.

2. In a food processor, add the bulgur, beef, shallot, parsley, spices, salt, and pulse until a smooth mixture is formed.
3. Situate the mixture into a bowl and refrigerate, covered for about 30 minutes. Remove from the refrigerator and make equal sized balls from the beef mixture.
4. In a large nonstick skillet, heat the oil over medium-high heat and cook the meatballs in 2 batches for about 13-14 minutes, flipping frequently. Serve warm.

NUTRITION: 228 Calories 7.4g Fat 0.1g Carbohydrates 3.5g Protein 766mg Sodium

Tasty Beef and Broccoli

Preparation Time: 10 minutes

Cooking Time: **15 minutes**

Servings: **2**

INGREDIENTS:

- 1 and ½ lbs. flanks steak
- 1 tbsp. olive oil
- 1 tbsp. tamari sauce
- 1 cup beef stock
- 1-pound broccoli, florets separated

DIRECTIONS:

1. Combine steak strips with oil and tamari, toss and set aside for 10 minutes. Select your instant pot on sauté mode, place beef strips and brown them for 4 minutes on each side.
2. Stir in stock, cover the pot again and cook on high for 8 minutes. Stir in broccoli, cover and cook on high for 4 minutes more.
3. Portion everything between plates and serve. Enjoy!

NUTRITION: 312 Calories 5g Fat 20g Carbohydrates 4g Protein 694mg Sodium

Soy Sauce Beef Roast

Preparation Time: 8 minutes
Cooking Time: 35 minutes
Servings: 2

INGREDIENTS:

- ½ teaspoon beef bouillon
- 1 ½ teaspoon rosemary
- ½ teaspoon minced garlic
- 2 pounds roast beef
- 1/3 cup soy sauce

DIRECTIONS:

1. Combine the soy sauce, bouillon, rosemary, and garlic together in a mixing bowl.
2. Turn on your instant pot. Place the roast, and pour enough water to cover the roast; gently stir to mix well. Seal it tight.
3. Click "MEAT/STEW" Cooking function; set pressure level to "HIGH" and set the Cooking time to 35 minutes. Let the pressure to build to cook the ingredients. Once done, click "CANCEL" setting then click "NPR" Cooking function to release the pressure naturally.

4. Gradually open the lid, and shred the meat. Mix in the shredded meat back in the potting mix and stir well. Transfer in serving containers. Serve warm.

NUTRITION: 423 Calories 14g Fat 12g Carbohydrates 21g Protein 884mg Sodium

Mediterranean Grilled Pork Chops

Preparation time: 1 day & 15 minutes

Cooking time: 20 minutes

Servings: 6

INGREDIENTS:

- ✓ 2 pork chops
- ✓ ¼ cup olive oil
- ✓ 2 yellow onions, sliced
- ✓ 2 garlic cloves, minced
- ✓ 2 teaspoons mustard
- ✓ 1 teaspoon sweet paprika
- ✓ Salt and black pepper to taste
- ✓ ½ teaspoon oregano, dried
- ✓ ½ teaspoon thyme, dried
- ✓ A pinch of cayenne pepper

DIRECTIONS:

1. In a small bowl, mix oil with garlic, mustard, paprika, black pepper, oregano, thyme and cayenne and whisk well.
2. In a bowl, combine onions with meat and mustard mix, toss to coat, cover and keep in the fridge for 1 day.

3. Place meat on preheated grill pan over medium high heat, season with salt and cook for 10 minutes on each side.
4. Meanwhile, heat a pan over medium heat, add marinated onions, stir and sauté for 4 minutes. Divide pork chops on plates, add sautéed onions on top and serve.

NUTRITION: Calories 234 Fat 3g Carbs 21g Protein 23g

Simple Pork Stir Fry

Preparation time: 10 minutes
Cooking time: 15 minutes
Servings: 4

INGREDIENTS:

- ✓ 4 ounces bacon, chopped
- ✓ 4 ounces snow peas
- ✓ 2 tablespoons butter
- ✓ 1-pound pork loin, cut into thin strips
- ✓ 2 cups mushrooms, sliced
- ✓ ¾ cup white wine
- ✓ ½ cup yellow onion, chopped
- ✓ 3 tablespoons sour cream
- ✓ Salt and white pepper to taste

DIRECTIONS:

1. Put snow peas in a saucepan, add water to cover, add a pinch of salt, bring to a boil over medium heat, cook until they are soft, drain and leave aside.
2. Heat a pan over medium high heat, add bacon, cook for a few minutes, drain grease, transfer to a bowl and leave aside.

3. Heat a pan with 1 tablespoon butter over medium heat, add pork strips, salt and pepper to taste, brown for a few minutes and transfer to a plate as well.
4. Return pan to medium heat, add remaining butter and melt it. Add onions and mushrooms, stir and cook for 4 minutes.
5. Add wine, and simmer until it's reduced. Add cream, peas, pork, salt and pepper to taste, stir, heat up, divide between plates, top with bacon and serve.

NUTRITION: Calories 343 Fat 31g Carbs 21g Protein 23g

Pork and Lentil Soup

Preparation time: 10 minutes
Cooking time: 1 hour
Servings: 6

INGREDIENTS:

- ✓ 1 small yellow onion, chopped
- ✓ 1 tablespoon olive oil
- ✓ 1 and ½ teaspoons basil, chopped
- ✓ 1 and ½ teaspoons ginger, grated
- ✓ 3 garlic cloves, chopped
- ✓ Salt and black pepper to taste
- ✓ ½ teaspoon cumin, ground
- ✓ 1 carrot, chopped
- ✓ 1-pound pork chops, bone-in 3 ounces brown lentils, rinsed
- ✓ 3 cups chicken stock
- ✓ 2 tablespoons tomato paste
- ✓ 2 tablespoons lime juice
- ✓ 1 teaspoon red chili flakes, crushed

DIRECTIONS:

1. Heat a saucepan with the oil over medium heat, add garlic, onion, basil, ginger, salt, pepper and cumin, stir well and cook for 6 minutes.
2. Add carrots, stir and cook 5 more minutes. Add pork and brown for a few minutes. Add lentils, tomato paste and stock, stir, bring to a boil, cover pan and simmer for 50 minutes.
3. Transfer pork to a plate, discard bones, shred it and return to pan. Add chili flakes and lime juice, stir, ladle into bowls and serve.

NUTRITION: Calories 343 Fat 31g Carbs 21g Protein 23g

Simple Braised Pork

Preparation time: 40 minutes
Cooking time: 1 hour
Servings: 4
INGREDIENTS:

- ✓ 2 pounds pork loin roast, boneless and cubed
- ✓ 5 tablespoons butter
- ✓ Salt and black pepper to taste
- ✓ 2 cups chicken stock
- ✓ ½ cup dry white wine
- ✓ 2 garlic cloves, minced
- ✓ 1 teaspoon thyme, chopped
- ✓ 1 thyme spring
- ✓ 1 bay leaf
- ✓ ½ yellow onion, chopped
- ✓ 2 tablespoons white flour
- ✓ ¾ pound pearl onions
- ✓ ½ pound red grapes

DIRECTIONS:

1. Heat a pan with 2 tablespoons butter over high heat, add pork loin, some salt and pepper, stir, brown for 10 minutes and transfer to a plate.
2. Add wine to the pan, bring to a boil over high heat and cook for 3 minutes.
3. Add stock, garlic, thyme spring, bay leaf, yellow onion and return meat to the pan, bring to a boil, cover, reduce heat to low, cook for 1 hour, strain liquid into another saucepan and transfer pork to a plate.
4. Put pearl onions in a small saucepan, add water to cover, bring to a boil over medium high heat, boil them for 5 minutes, drain, peel them and leave aside for now.
5. In a bowl, mix 2 tablespoons butter with flour and stir well. Add ½ cup of strained cooking liquid and whisk well.
6. Pour this into cooking liquid, bring to a simmer over medium heat and cook for 5 minutes. Add salt and pepper, chopped thyme, pork and pearl onions, cover and simmer for a few minutes.
7. Meanwhile, heat a pan with 1 tablespoon butter, add grapes, stir and cook them for 1-2 minutes.

Divide pork meat on plates, drizzle the sauce all over and serve with onions and grapes on the side.

NUTRITION: Calories 320 Fat 31g Carbs 21g Protein 23g

Pork and Chickpea Stew

Preparation time: 20 minutes
Cooking time: 8 hours
Servings: 4

INGREDIENTS:

- ✓ 2 tablespoons white flour
- ✓ ½ cup chicken stock
- ✓ 1 tablespoon ginger, grated
- ✓ 1 teaspoon coriander, ground
- ✓ 2 teaspoons cumin, ground
- ✓ Salt and black pepper to taste
- ✓ 2 and ½ pounds pork butt, cubed
- ✓ 28 ounces canned tomatoes, drained and chopped
- ✓ 4 ounces carrots, chopped
- ✓ 1 red onion cut in wedges
- ✓ 4 garlic cloves, minced
- ✓ ½ cup apricots, cut in quarters
- ✓ 1 cup couscous, cooked
- ✓ 15 ounces canned chickpeas, drained
- ✓ Cilantro, chopped for serving

DIRECTIONS:

1. Put stock in your slow cooker. Add flour, cumin, ginger, coriander, salt and pepper and stir. Add tomatoes, pork, carrots, garlic, onion and apricots, cover cooker and cook on Low for 7 hours and 50 minutes.
2. Add chickpeas and couscous, cover and cook for 10 more minutes. Divide on plates, sprinkle cilantro and serve right away.

NUTRITION: Calories 216 Fat 31g Carbs 21g Protein 23g

Pork and Greens Salad

Preparation time: 10 minutes
Cooking time: 15 minutes
Servings: 4

INGREDIENTS:

- ✓ 1-pound pork chops, boneless and cut into strips
- ✓ 8 ounces white mushrooms, sliced
- ✓ ½ cup Italian dressing
- ✓ 6 cups mixed salad greens
- ✓ 6 ounces jarred artichoke hearts, drained
- ✓ Salt and black pepper to the taste
- ✓ ½ cup basil, chopped
- ✓ 1 tablespoon olive oil

DIRECTIONS:

1. Heat a pan with the oil over medium-high heat, add the pork and brown for 5 minutes. Add the mushrooms, stir and sauté for 5 minutes more.
2. Add the dressing, artichokes, salad greens, salt, pepper and the basil, cook for 4-5 minutes, divide everything into bowls and serve.

NUTRITION: Calories 320 Fat 31g Carbs 21g Protein 23g

Pork Strips and Rice

Preparation time: 10 minutes
Cooking time: 25 minutes
Servings: 4

INGREDIENTS:

- ½ pound pork loin, cut into strips
- Salt and black pepper to taste
- 2 tablespoons olive oil
- 2 carrots, chopped
- 1 red bell pepper, chopped
- 3 garlic cloves, minced
- 2 cups veggie stock
- 1 cup basmati rice
- ½ cup garbanzo beans
- 10 black olives, pitted and sliced
- 1 tablespoon parsley, chopped

DIRECTIONS:

1. Heat a pan with the oil over medium high heat. Add the pork fillets, stir, cook for 5 minutes and transfer them to a plate.
2. Add the carrots, bell pepper and the garlic, stir and cook for 5 more minutes.

3. Add the rice, the stock, beans and the olives, stir, cook for 14 minutes, divide between plates, sprinkle the parsley on top and serve.

NUTRITION: Calories 220 Fat 31g Carbs 21g Protein 23g

Slow Cooked Mediterranean Pork

Preparation time: 20 hours and 10 minutes

Cooking time: 8 hours

Servings: 6

INGREDIENTS:

- ✓ 3 pounds pork shoulder - boneless
- ✓ ¼ cup olive oil
- ✓ 2 teaspoons oregano, dried
- ✓ ¼ cup lemon juice
- ✓ 2 teaspoons mustard
- ✓ 2 teaspoons mint, chopped
- ✓ 3 garlic cloves, minced
- ✓ 2 teaspoons pesto sauce
- ✓ Salt and black pepper to taste

DIRECTIONS:

1. In a bowl, mix olive oil with lemon juice, oregano, mint, mustard, garlic, pesto, salt and pepper then whisk well.
2. Rub pork with marinade, cover and keep in a cold place for 10 hours. Flip pork shoulder and leave aside for 10 more hours.

3. Transfer to your slow cooker along with the marinade juices, cover and cook on low for 8 hours. Uncover, slice, divide between plates and serve.

NUTRITION: Calories 320 Fat 31g Carbs 21g Protein 23g

Pork and Bean Stew

Preparation time: 20 minutes
Cooking time: 4 hours
Servings: 4

INGREDIENTS:

- ✓ 2 pounds pork neck
- ✓ 1 tablespoon white flour
- ✓ 1 and ½ tablespoons olive oil
- ✓ 2 eggplants, chopped
- ✓ 1 brown onion, chopped
- ✓ 1 red bell pepper, chopped
- ✓ 3 garlic cloves, minced
- ✓ 1 tablespoon thyme, dried
- ✓ 2 teaspoons sage, dried
- ✓ 4 ounces canned white beans, drained
- ✓ 1 cup chicken stock
- ✓ 12 ounces zucchinis, chopped
- ✓ Salt and pepper to taste
- ✓ 2 tablespoons tomato paste

DIRECTIONS:

1. In a bowl, mix flour with salt, pepper, pork neck and toss. Heat a pan with 2 teaspoons oil over medium high heat, add pork and cook for 3 minutes on each side.
2. Transfer pork to a slow cooker and leave aside. Heat the remaining oil in the same pan over medium heat, add eggplant, onion, bell pepper, thyme, sage and garlic, stir and cook for 5 minutes.
3. Add reserved flour, stir and cook for 1 more minute. Add to pork, then add beans, stock, tomato paste and zucchinis. Cover and cook on high for 4 hours. Uncover, transfer to plates and serve.

NUTRITION: Calories: 310 fat 31g carbs 21g protein 23g

Pork with Couscous

Preparation time: 10 minutes
Cooking time: 7 hours
Servings: 6

INGREDIENTS:

- ✓ 2 and ½ pounds pork loin boneless and trimmed
- ✓ ¾ cup chicken stock
- ✓ 2 tablespoons olive oil
- ✓ ½ tablespoon sweet paprika
- ✓ 2 and ¼ teaspoon sage, dried
- ✓ ½ tablespoon garlic powder
- ✓ ¼ teaspoon rosemary, dried
- ✓ ¼ teaspoon marjoram, dried
- ✓ 1 teaspoon basil, dried
- ✓ 1 teaspoon oregano, dried
- ✓ Salt and black pepper to taste
- ✓ 2 cups couscous, cooked

DIRECTIONS:

- In a bowl, mix oil with stock, paprika, garlic powder, sage, rosemary, thyme, marjoram, oregano, salt and pepper to taste and whisk well. Put pork loin in your crock pot.

- Add stock and spice mix, stir, cover and cook on Low for 7 hours. Slice pork return to pot and toss with cooking juices. Divide between plates and serve with couscous on the side.

NUTRITION: Calories 320 Fat 31g Carbs 21g Protein 23g

Grilled Steak, Mushroom, and Onion Kebabs

Preparation Time: 10 minutes
Cooking Time: 10 minutes
Servings: 2
INGREDIENTS:

- Boneless top sirloin steak, 1 lb.
- White button mushrooms, 8 oz.
- Medium red onion, 1.
- Peeled garlic cloves, 4.
- Rosemary sprigs, 2.
- Extra-virgin olive oil, 2 tbsp.
- Black pepper, ¼ tsp.
- Red wine vinegar, 2 tbsp.
- Sea salt, ¼ tsp.

DIRECTIONS:

1. Soak 12 (10-inch) wooden skewers in water. Spray the cold grill with nonstick cooking spray, and heat the grill to medium-high.
2. Cut a piece of aluminum foil into a 10-inch square. Place the garlic and rosemary sprigs in

the center, drizzle with 1 tablespoon of oil, and wrap tightly to form a foil packet.
3. Arrange it on the grill, and seal the grill cover.
4. Cut the steak into 1-inch cubes. Thread the beef onto the wet skewers, alternating with whole mushrooms and onion wedges. Spray the kebabs thoroughly with nonstick cooking spray, and sprinkle with pepper.
5. Cook the kebabs on the covered grill for 5 minutes.
6. Flip and grill for 5 more minutes while covered.
7. Unwrap foil packets with garlic and rosemary sprigs and put them into a small bowl.
8. Carefully strip the rosemary sprigs of their leaves into the bowl and pour in any accumulated juices and oil from the foil packet.
9. Mix in the remaining 1 tablespoon of oil and the vinegar and salt.Mash the garlic with a fork, and mix all ingredients in the bowl together. Pour over the finished steak kebabs and serve.

NUTRITION: Calories: 410, Protein: 36 g, Carbohydrates: 12 g, Fat: 14 g

Turkey Meatballs

Preparation Time: 10 minutes
Cooking Time: 25 minutes
Servings: 2

INGREDIENTS:

- ✓ Diced yellow onion, ¼
- ✓ Diced artichoke hearts, 14 oz.
- ✓ Ground turkey, 1 lb.
- ✓ Dried parsley, 1 tsp.
- ✓ Oil, 1 tsp.
- ✓ Chopped basil, 4 tbsp.
- ✓ Pepper and salt, to taste.

DIRECTIONS:

1. Grease the baking sheet and preheat the oven to 3500 F.
2. On medium heat, place a nonstick medium saucepan, sauté artichoke hearts, and diced onions for 5 minutes or until onions are soft.
3. Meanwhile, in a big bowl, mix parsley, basil and ground turkey with hands. Season to taste.
4. Once onion mixture has cooled, add into the bowl and mix thoroughly.

5. With an ice cream scooper, scoop ground turkey and form balls.
6. Place on a prepared cooking sheet, pop in the oven and bake until cooked around 15-20 minutes.
7. Remove from pan, serve and enjoy

NUTRITION: Calories: 283, Protein: 12 g, Carbohydrates: 30 g, Fat: 12 g

Chicken Marsala

Preparation Time: 10 minutes

Cooking Time: 45 minutes

Servings: 2

INGREDIENTS:

- ✓ 2 tablespoons olive oil
- ✓ 4 skinless, boneless chicken breast cutlets
- ✓ ¾ tablespoons black pepper, divided
- ✓ ½ teaspoon kosher salt, divided
- ✓ 8 oz. mushrooms, sliced
- ✓ 4 thyme sprigs
- ✓ 0.2 quarts unsalted chicken stock
- ✓ quarts Marsala wine
- ✓ tablespoons olive oil
- ✓ tablespoon fresh thyme, chopped

DIRECTIONS:

1. Heat oil in a pan and fry chicken for 4-5 minutes per side. Remove chicken from the pan and set it aside.
2. In same pan add thyme, mushrooms, salt, and pepper; stir fry for 1-2 minutes.

3. Add Marsala wine, chicken broth, and cooked chicken. Let simmer for 10-12 minutes on low heat.
4. Add to a serving dish.
5. Enjoy.

NUTRITION: Calories – 206, Fat –17 g, Carbs – 3 g, Protein – 8 g

Cauliflower Steaks with Eggplant Relish

Preparation Time: 5 minutes

Cooking Time: 25 minutes

Servings: 2

INGREDIENTS:

- ✓ 2 small heads cauliflower (about 3 pounds)
- ✓ ¼ teaspoon kosher or sea salt
- ✓ ¼ teaspoon smoked paprika
- ✓ Extra-virgin olive oil, divided

DIRECTIONS:

1. Place a large, rimmed baking sheet in the oven. Preheat the oven to 400°F with the pan inside.
2. Stand one head of cauliflower on a cutting board, stem-end down. With a long chef's knife, slice down through the very center of the head, including the stem.
3. Starting at the cut edge, measure about 1 inch and cut one thick slice from each cauliflower half, including as much of the stem as possible, to make two cauliflower "steaks."
4. Reserve the remaining cauliflower for another use. Repeat with the second cauliflower head.

5. Dry each steak well with a clean towel. Sprinkle the salt and smoked paprika evenly over both sides of each cauliflower steak.
6. In a large skillet over medium-high heat, heat 2 tablespoons of oil. When the oil is very hot, add two cauliflower steaks to the pan and cook for about 3 minutes, until golden and crispy. Flip and cook for 2 more minutes.
7. Transfer the steaks to a plate. Use a pair of tongs to hold a paper towel and wipe out the pan to remove most of the hot oil (which will contain a few burnt bits of cauliflower).
8. Repeat the cooking process with the remaining 2 tablespoons of oil and the remaining two steaks.
9. Using oven mitts, carefully remove the baking sheet from the oven and place the cauliflower on the baking sheet. Roast in the oven for 12 to 15 minutes, until the cauliflower steaks are just fork tender; they will still be somewhat firm. Serve the steaks with the Eggplant Relish Spread, baba ghanoush, or the homemade ketchup.

NUTRITION: Calories – 206, Fat –17 g, Carbs – 3 g, Protein – 8 g

Lemon Caper Chicken

Preparation Time: 10 minutes

Cooking Time: 15 minutes

Servings: 2

INGREDIENTS:

- ✓ 2 tablespoon virgin olive oil
- ✓ 2 chicken breasts (boneless, skinless, cut in half, pound to ¾ an inch thick)
- ✓ ¼ cup capers
- ✓ 2 lemons (wedges)
- ✓ 1 teaspoon oregano
- ✓ 1 teaspoon basil
- ✓ ½ teaspoon black pepper

DIRECTIONS:

1. Take a large skillet and place it on your stove and add the olive oil to it. Turn the heat to medium and allow it to warm up.
2. As the oil heats up season your chicken breast with the oregano, basil, and black pepper on each side.
3. Place your chicken breast into the hot skillet and cook on each side for five minutes.

4. Transfer the chicken from the skillet to your dinner plate. Top with capers and serve with a few lemon wedges.

NUTRITION: Calories – 182, Carbs - 3.4 g, Protein - 26.6 g, Fat - 8.2 g

Herb Roasted Chicken

Preparation Time: 20 minutes
Cooking Time: 45 minutes
Servings: 2

INGREDIENTS:

- ✓ 1 tablespoon virgin olive oil
- ✓ 1 whole chicken
- ✓ 2 rosemary springs
- ✓ 3 garlic cloves (peeled)
- ✓ 1 lemon (cut in half)
- ✓ 1 teaspoon sea salt
- ✓ 1 teaspoon black pepper

DIRECTIONS:

1. Turn your oven to 450 degrees F.
2. Take your whole chicken and pat it dry using paper towels. Then rub in the olive oil. Remove the leaves from one of the springs of rosemary and scatter them over the chicken. Sprinkle the sea salt and black pepper over top. Place the other whole sprig of rosemary into the cavity of the chicken. Then add in the garlic cloves and lemon halves.

3. Place the chicken into a roasting pan and then place it into the oven. Allow the chicken to bake for 1 hour, then check that the internal temperature should be at least 165 degrees F. If the chicken begins to brown too much, cover it with foil and return it to the oven to finish cooking.
4. When the chicken has cooked to the appropriate temperature remove it from the oven. Let it rest for at least 20 minutes before carving.
5. Serve with a large side of roasted or steamed vegetables or your favorite salad.

NUTRITION: Calories – 309, Carbs - 1.5 g, Protein - 27.2 g, Fat - 21.3 g

Mediterranean bowl

Preparation Time: 25 minutes
Cooking Time: 30 minutes
Servings: 2
INGREDIENTS:

- ✓ 2 chicken breasts (chopped into 4 halves)
- ✓ 2 diced onions
- ✓ 2 bottles of lemon pepper marinade
- ✓ 2 diced green bell pepper
- ✓ 4 lemon juices
- ✓ 8 cloves of crushed garlic.
- ✓ 5 teaspoon of olive oil
- ✓ Feta cheese
- ✓ 1 grape tomato
- ✓ 1 large-sized diced zucchini and 1 small-sized. Otherwise, use two medium-sized diced zucchinis.
- ✓ Salt and pepper (according to your desired taste), 4 cups of water.
- ✓ Kalamata olives (as much as you fancy)
- ✓ 1 cup of garbanzo beans

NUTRITION: 541 Cal, 34g of protein, 1423mg of potassium, 12g of fiber, 15g of sugar, 72mg of cholesterol, 4g of fat, 45g of carbs.

Tasty Lamb Leg

Preparation Time: 10 minutes

Cooking Time: 20 minutes

Servings: 2

INGREDIENTS:

- ✓ 2 lbs. leg of lamb, boneless and cut into chunks
- ✓ 1 tbsp. olive oil
- ✓ 1 tbsp. garlic, sliced
- ✓ 1 cup red wine
- ✓ 1 cup onion, chopped
- ✓ 2 carrots, chopped
- ✓ 1 tsp. rosemary, chopped
- ✓ 2 tsp. thyme, chopped
- ✓ 1 tsp. oregano, chopped
- ✓ 1/2 cup beef stock
- ✓ 2 tbsp. tomato paste
- ✓ Pepper
- ✓ Salt

DIRECTIONS:

- Add oil into the inner pot of instant pot and set the pot on sauté mode.

- Add meat and sauté until browned.
- Add remaining ingredients and stir well.
- Seal pot with lid and cook on high for 15 minutes.
- Once done, allow to release pressure naturally. Remove lid.
- Stir well and serve.

NUTRITION: Calories 540, Fat 20.4 g, Carbohydrates 10.3 g, Sugar 4.2 g, Protein 65.2 g, Cholesterol 204 mg

Kale Sprouts & Lamb

Preparation Time: 10 minutes
Cooking Time: 30 minutes
Servings: 2
INGREDIENTS:

- ✓ 2 lbs. lamb, cut into chunks
- ✓ 1 tbsp. parsley, chopped
- ✓ 2 tbsp. olive oil
- ✓ 1 cup kale, chopped
- ✓ 1 cup Brussels sprouts, halved
- ✓ 1 cup beef stock
- ✓ Pepper
- ✓ Salt

DIRECTIONS:

- Add all ingredients into the inner pot of instant pot and stir well.
- Seal pot with lid and cook on high for 30 minutes.
- Once done, allow to release pressure naturally. Remove lid.
- Serve and enjoy.

NUTRITION: Calories 504, Fat 23.8 g, Carbohydrates 3.9 g, Sugar 0.5 g, Protein 65.7 g, Cholesterol 204 mg

Grilled Harissa Chicken

Preparation Time: 20 minutes

Cooking Time: 12 minutes

Servings: 2

INGREDIENTS:

- ✓ Juice of 1 lemon
- ✓ 1/2 sliced red onion
- ✓ 1 ½ teaspoon of coriander
- ✓ 1 ½ teaspoon of smoked paprika
- ✓ 1 teaspoon of cumin
- ✓ 2 teaspoons of cayenne
- ✓ Olive oil
- ✓ 1 ½ teaspoon of Black pepper
- ✓ Kosher salt
- ✓ 5 ounces of thawed and drained frozen spinach
- ✓ 8 boneless chickens.

DIRECTIONS:

1. Get a large bowl. Season your chicken with kosher salt on all sides, then add onions, garlic, lemon juice, and harissa paste to the bowl.

2. Add about 3 tablespoons of olive oil to the mixture. Heat a grill to 459 heat (an indoor or outdoor grill works just fine), then oil the grates.
3. Grill each side of the chicken for about 7 minutes. Its temperature should register 165 degrees on a thermometer and it should be fully cooked by then.

NUTRITION: 142.5 kcal, 4.7g of fat, 1.2g of saturated fat, 102mg of sodium, 1.7g of carbs, 107.4mg of cholesterol, 22.1g of protein.

Italian Chicken Meatballs

Preparation Time: 20 minutes
Cooking Time: 32 minutes
Servings: 20
INGREDIENTS:

- ✓ 3 tomatoes
- ✓ Kosher salt
- ✓ ½ cup of freshly chopped parsley
- ✓ 1 teaspoon of dry oregano
- ✓ Kosher salt
- ✓ ½ teaspoon of fresh thyme
- ✓ ¼ teaspoon of sweet paprika
- ✓ 1 red onion
- ✓ 1 lb. of ground chicken
- ✓ ½ minced garlic cloves
- ✓ Black pepper
- ✓ 1 raw egg
- ✓ ¼ cup of freshly grated parmesan cheese
- ✓ Extra virgin olive oil.

DIRECTIONS:

1. Heat the oven to 375 degrees and get a cooking pan. Coat with extra virgin olive oil and set aside.
2. Get a large bowl and mix your tomatoes with kosher salt and thinly chopped onions.
3. Add half of your fresh thyme and sprinkle a little extra virgin olive oil on it again.
4. Transfer this to your cooking and use a spoon to spread. Add ground chicken to the mixing bowl you recently used, and add egg, parmesan cheese and oregano.
5. Include paprika, garlic, the other half of thyme, chopped parsley and black pepper.
6. Sprinkle a little amount of extra virgin olive oil on it, and mix till the meatball mixture is combined. Form about 1 ½ inch chicken meatballs with the mixture and cut it all to this size.
7. Get another cooking pan and arrange these meatballs in it. Add tomatoes and onions, and blend them with the meatballs. Bake in your preheated oven for about 30 min.
8. Your meatballs should turn golden brown, you can make them more colorful by removing them and

coating them with extra virgin olive oil before you continue baking.

9. But that is not necessary. A couple of minutes after this, your meatballs cam is served. No surprises, your tomatoes are fast falling.

NUTRITION: 79 kcal, 74.7mg of sodium, 1.4g of sugar, 301.1g of potassium, 0.92g of fiber, 44.2mg of calcium, 0.94g of iron, 4.1g of carbs, 7.8g of protein.

Classic Chicken Cooking with Tomatoes & Tapenade

Preparation Time: 25 minutes
Cooking Time: 25 minutes
Servings: 2
INGREDIENTS:

- ✓ 4-5 oz. chicken breasts, boneless and skinless
- ✓ ¼-tsp salt (divided)
- ✓ 3-tbsp fresh basil leaves, chopped (divided)
- ✓ 1-tbsp olive oil
- ✓ 1½-cups cherry tomatoes, halved
- ✓ ¼-cup olive tapenade

DIRECTIONS:

1. Arrange the chicken on a sheet of glassine or waxed paper. Sprinkle half of the salt and a third of the basil evenly over the chicken.
2. Press lightly, and flip over the chicken pieces. Sprinkle the remaining salt and another third of the basil. Cover the seasoned chicken with another sheet of waxed paper.
3. By using a meat mallet or rolling pin, pound the chicken to a half-inch thickness.

4. Heat the olive oil in a 12-inch skillet placed over medium-high heat. Add the pounded chicken breasts.
5. Cook for 6 minutes on each side until the chicken turns golden brown with no traces of pink in the middle. Transfer the browned chicken breasts in a platter, and cover to keep them warm.
6. In the same skillet, add the olive tapenade and tomatoes. Cook for 3 minutes until the tomatoes just begin to be tender.
7. To serve, pour over the tomato-tapenade mixture over the cooked chicken breasts, and top with the remaining basil.

NUTRITION: Calories: 190, Fats: 7g, Dietary Fiber: 1g, Carbohydrates: 6g, Protein: 26g

Turkish Turkey Mini Meatloaves

Preparation Time: 15 minutes
Cooking Time: 20 minutes
Servings: 2
INGREDIENTS:

- ✓ 1-lb. ground turkey breast
- ✓ 1-pc egg
- ✓ ¼-cup whole-wheat breadcrumbs, crushed
- ✓ ¼-cup feta cheese, plus more for topping
- ✓ ¼-cup Kalamata olives, halved
- ✓ ¼-cup fresh parsley, chopped
- ✓ ¼-cup red onion, minced
- ✓ ¼-cup + 2-tbsp hummus
- ✓ 2-cloves garlic, minced
- ✓ ½-tsp dried basil
- ✓ ¼- tsp. dried oregano
- ✓ Salt & pepper
- ✓ ½-pc small cucumber, peeled, seeded, and chopped
- ✓ 1-pc large tomato, chopped
- ✓ 3-tbsp fresh basil, chopped

- ✓ ½-lemon, juice
- ✓ 1-tsp extra-virgin olive oil
- ✓ Salt & pepper

DIRECTIONS:

- Preheat your oven to 425 °F.
- Line a 5"x9" baking sheet with foil, and spray the surfaces with non-stick grease. Set aside.
- Except for the ¼-cup hummus, combine and mix all the turkey meatloaf ingredients in a large mixing bowl. Mix well until fully combined.
- Divide mixture equally into 4 portions. Form the portions into loaves. Spread a tablespoon of the remaining hummus on each meatloaf. Place the loaves on the greased baking sheet.
- Bake for 20 minutes until the loaves no longer appear pink in the center. (Ensure the meatloaf cooks through by inserting a meat thermometer and the reading reaches 165 °F.)
- Combine and mix all the topping ingredients in a small mixing bowl. Mix well until fully combined.
- To serve, spoon the topping over the cooked meatloaves.

NUTRITION: Calories: 130, Fats: 7g, Dietary Fiber: 4g, Carbohydrates: 14g, Protein: 6g

Charred Chicken Souvlaki Skewers

Preparation Time: 20 minutes

Cooking Time: 15 minutes

Servings: 2

INGREDIENTS:

- ✓ ½-cup olive oil
- ✓ ½-cup fresh squeezed lemon juice
- ✓ 1-tbsp red wine vinegar
- ✓ 1-tbsp finely minced garlic (or garlic puree from a jar)
- ✓ 1-tbsp dried Greek oregano
- ✓ 1-tsp dried thyme
- ✓ 6-pcs chicken breasts, boneless, skinless, with trimmed off tendons and fats
- ✓ Fresh cucumber and cherry tomatoes for garnish

DIRECTIONS:

- Combine and mix all the marinade ingredients in a small mixing bowl. Mix well until fully combined.
- Slice each chicken breast crosswise into six 1-inch strips.
- Place the chicken strips into a large plastic container with a tight-fitting lid.

- Pour the marinade into the plastic container, and seal with its lid. Gently shake the container and turn it over so that the marinade evenly coats all of the meat. Refrigerate the sealed plastic container to marinate for 8 hours or more.
- Spray the grill's surfaces with non-stick grease. Preheat your charcoal or gas barbecue grill to medium-high heat.
- Take the chicken out and let it cool to room temperature. Drain the chicken pieces and thread them onto skewers. (Try to thread six pieces for each skewer and fold over each chicken piece so it will not spin around the skewer.)
- Grill the chicken souvlaki skewers for 15 minutes, turning once after seeing the appearance of desirable grill marks.
- To serve, place the souvlaki on a serving plate alongside the cucumber and tomato garnish.

NUTRITION: Calories: 360, Fats: 26g, Dietary Fiber: 0g, Carbohydrates: 3g, Protein: 30g

Mediterranean Lamb Chops

Preparation Time: 10 minutes
Cooking Time: 10 minutes
Servings: 2

INGREDIENTS:

- ✓ 4 lamb shoulder chops, 8 ounces each
- ✓ 2 tablespoons Dijon mustard
- ✓ 2 tablespoons Balsamic vinegar
- ✓ 1 tablespoon garlic, chopped
- ✓ ½ cup olive oil
- ✓ 2 tablespoons shredded fresh basil

DIRECTIONS:

1. Pat your lamb chop dry using a kitchen towel and arrange them on a shallow glass baking dish.
2. Take a bowl and whisk in Dijon mustard, balsamic vinegar, garlic, pepper, and mix well.
3. Whisk in the oil very slowly into the marinade until the mixture is smooth.
4. Stir in basil.
5. Pour the marinade over the lamb chops and stir to coat both sides well.
6. Cover the chops and allow them to marinate for 1-4 hours (chilled).

7. Take the chops out and leave them for 30 minutes to allow the temperature to reach the normal level.
8. Preheat your grill to medium heat and add oil to the grate.
9. Grill the lamb chops for 5-10 minutes per side until both sides are browned. Once the center of the chop reads 145-degree Fahrenheit, the chops are ready, serve and enjoy!

Nutrition: Calories: 521, Fat: 45g, Carbs: 3.5g, Protein: 22g

Mushroom and Beef Risotto

Preparation Time: 5 minutes

Cooking Time: 10 minutes

Servings: 2

INGREDIENTS:

- ✓ 2 cups low-sodium beef stock
- ✓ 2 cups water
- ✓ 2 tablespoon olive oil
- ✓ ½ cup scallions, chopped
- ✓ 1 cup Arborio rice
- ✓ ¼ cup dry white wine
- ✓ 1 cup roast beef, thinly stripped
- ✓ 1 cup button mushrooms
- ✓ ½ cup canned cream of mushroom
- ✓ Salt and pepper as needed
- ✓ Oregano, chopped
- ✓ Parsley, chopped

DIRECTIONS:

1. Take a stock pot and put it over medium heat.
2. Add water with beef stock in it.
3. Bring the mixture to a boil and remove the heat.

4. Take another heavy-bottomed saucepan and put it over medium heat.
5. Add in the scallions and stir fry them for 1 minute.
6. Add in the rice then and cook it for at least 2 minutes, occasionally stirring it to ensure that it is finely coated with oil.
7. In the rice mixture, keep adding your beef stock ½ a cup at a time, making sure to stir it often.
8. Once all the stock has been added, cook the rice for another 2 minutes.
9. During the last 5 minutes of your cooking, make sure to add the beef, cream of mushroom while stirring it nicely.   Transfer the whole mix to a serving dish. Garnish with some chopped up parsley and oregano. Serve hot.

NUTRITION: Calories: 378, Fat: 12g, Carbs: 41g, Protein: 23g

Oven Roasted Garlic Chicken Thigh

Preparation time: 10 minutes
Cooking time: 55 minutes
Servings: 2
INGREDIENTS:

- ✓ 8 chicken thighs
- ✓ Salt and pepper as needed
- ✓ 1 tablespoon extra-virgin olive oil
- ✓ 6 cloves garlic, peeled and crushed
- ✓ 1 jar (10 ounces) roasted red peppers, drained and chopped
- ✓ 1 1/2 pounds potatoes, diced
- ✓ 2 cups cherry tomatoes, halved
- ✓ 1/3 cup capers, sliced
- ✓ 1 teaspoon dried Italian seasoning
- ✓ 1 tablespoon fresh basil

DIRECTIONS:

1. Season chicken with kosher salt and black pepper.
2. Take a cast-iron skillet over medium-high heat and heat up olive oil.
3. Sear the chicken on both sides.

4. Add remaining ingredients except for basil and stir well.
5. Remove heat and place cast iron skillet in the oven.
6. Bake for 45 minutes at 400 degrees Fahrenheit until the internal temperature reaches 165 degrees Fahrenheit.
7. Serve and enjoy!

NUTRITION: Calories: 500, Fat: 23g, Carbs: 37g, Protein: 35g

Balearic Beef Brisket Bowl

Preparation Time: 0 minutes
Cooking Time: 50 minutes
Servings: 2

INGREDIENTS:

- ½-cup manto negro dry red wine (Spanish or Mallorca dry red wine)
- 1/3-cup olives, pitted and chopped
- 14.5-oz tomatoes with juice (diced)
- 5-cloves garlic, chopped
- ½-tsp dried rosemary
- Salt and pepper
- 2½-lbs. beef brisket
- Olive oil
- 1-tbsp fresh parsley, finely chopped
- 1½-cups sautéed green beans

DIRECTIONS:

1. Pour the dry wine and olives in your slow cooker, and stir in the tomatoes, garlic, and rosemary.
2. Sprinkle salt and pepper to taste over the beef brisket. Place the seasoned meat on top of the wine-tomato mixture. Ladle half of the mixture

over the meat. Cover the slow cooker, and cook for 6 hours on high heat until fork-tender.
3. Transfer the cooked brisket to a chopping board. Tent the meat with foil and let stand for 10 minutes.
4. Drizzle with olive oil. Cut the brisket into 6-slices across its grain. Transfer the slices in a serving platter, and spoon some sauce over the meat slices. Sprinkle with parsley.
5. Serve with sautéed green beans and the remaining sauce.

NUTRITION: Calories: 370, Fats: 18g, Dietary Fiber: 1g, Carbohydrates: 6g, Protein: 41g

Grilled Grapes & Chicken Chunks

Preparation Time: 15 minutes

Cooking Time: 30 minutes

Servings: 2

INGREDIENTS:

- ✓ 2-cloves garlic, minced
- ✓ ¼-cup extra-virgin olive oil
- ✓ 1-tbsp rosemary, minced
- ✓ 1-tbsp oregano, minced
- ✓ 1-tsp lemon zest
- ✓ ½-tsp red chili flakes, crushed
- ✓ 1-lb. chicken breast, boneless and skinless
- ✓ 1¾-cups green grapes, seedless and rinsed
- ✓ ½-tsp salt
- ✓ 1-tbsp lemon juice
- ✓ 2-tbsp extra-virgin olive oil

Directions:

1. Combine and mix all the marinade ingredients in a small mixing bowl. Mix well until fully combined. Set aside.

2. Cut the chicken breast into ¾-inch cubes. Alternately thread the chicken and grapes onto 12 skewers. Place the skewers in a large baking dish to hold them for marinating.
3. Pour the marinade over the skewers, coating them thoroughly. Marinate for 4 to 24 hours.
4. Remove the skewers from the marinade and allow dripping off any excess oil. Sprinkle over with salt.
5. Grill the chicken and grape skewers for 3 minutes on each side until cooked through.
6. To serve, arrange the skewers on a serving platter and drizzle with lemon juice and olive oil.

NUTRITION: Calories: 230, Fats: 20g, Dietary Fiber: 1g, Carbohydrates: 14g, Protein: 1g

Mediterranean Beef Skewers

Preparation Time: 5 minutes

Cooking Time: 8 minutes

Servings: 2

INGREDIENTS:

- ✓ Cubed beef sirloin, 2 lbs.
- ✓ Minced garlic cloves, 3
- ✓ Fresh lemon zest, 1 tbsp.
- ✓ Chopped parsley, 1 tbsp.
- ✓ Chopped thyme, 2 tsp.
- ✓ Minced rosemary, 2 tsp.
- ✓ Dried oregano, 2 tsp.
- ✓ Olive oil, 4 tbsp.
- ✓ Fresh lemon juice, 2 tbsp.
- ✓ Sea salt and ground black pepper, to taste

DIRECTIONS:

1. Add all the ingredients, except the beef, in a bowl.
2. Preheat the grill to medium-high heat.
3. Mix in the beef to marinate for 1 hour.
4. Arrange the marinated beef onto skewers then cook on the preheated grill for 8 minutes flipping occasionally.

5. Once cooked, leave aside to rest for 5 minutes then serve.

NUTRITION: Calories: 370, Protein: 60 g, Carbohydrates: 12 g, Fats: 46 g

Cumin Lamb Mix

Preparation time: 15 minutes
Cooking Time: 10 Minutes
Servings: 2

INGREDIENTS:

- ✓ 2 lamb chops (3.5 oz each)
- ✓ 1 tablespoon olive oil
- ✓ 1 teaspoon ground cumin
- ✓ ½ teaspoon salt

DIRECTIONS:

1. Rub the lamb chops with ground cumin and salt
2. Then sprinkle them with olive oil. Let the meat marinate for 10 minutes. After this, preheat the skillet well. Place the lamb chops in the skillet and roast them for 10 minutes. Flip the meat on another side from time to time to avoid burning.

NUTRITION: Calories 384 Fat 33.2g Carbs 0.5g Protein 19.2g

Beef & Potatoes

Preparation time: 15 minutes
Cooking Time: 20 Minutes
Servings: 6

INGREDIENTS:

- ✓ 1/2 lb. stew beef, sliced into cubes
- ✓ 2 teaspoons mixed dried herbs (thyme, sage)
- ✓ 4 potatoes, cubed
- ✓ 10 oz. mushrooms
- ✓ 1 ½ cups red wine

DIRECTIONS:

1. Set the Instant Pot to sauté. Add 1 tablespoon olive oil and cook the beef until brown on all sides. Add the rest of the ingredients.
2. Season with salt and pepper. Pour in 1 ½ cups water into the pot. Mix well. Cover the pot. Set it too manual. Cook at high pressure for 20 minutes. Release the pressure naturally.

NUTRITION: Calories 360 Fat 9.6g Carbohydrate 29.3g Protein 29.9g

Pork and Chestnuts Mix

Preparation time: 15 minutes

Cooking Time: 0 Minutes

Servings: 6

INGREDIENTS:

- ✓ **and ½ cups brown rice, already cooked**
- ✓ 2 cups pork roast, already cooked and shredded
- ✓ 3 ounces water chestnuts, drained and sliced
- ✓ ½ cup sour cream
- ✓ A pinch of salt and white pepper

DIRECTIONS:

1. In a bowl, mix the rice with the roast and the other ingredients, toss and keep in the fridge for 2 hours before serving.

NUTRITION: Calories 294 Fat 17g Carbs 16g Protein 23.5g

Rosemary Pork Chops

Preparation time: 15 minutes

Cooking Time: 25 Minutes

Servings: 4

INGREDIENTS:

- ✓ 4 pork loin chops, boneless
- ✓ Salt and black pepper to the taste
- ✓ 4 garlic cloves, minced
- ✓ 1 tablespoon rosemary, chopped
- ✓ 1 tablespoon olive oil

DIRECTIONS:

1. In a roasting pan, combine the pork chops with the rest of the ingredients, toss, and bake at 425 degrees F for 10 minutes.
2. Reduce the heat to 350 degrees F and cook the chops for 25 minutes more. Divide the chops between plates and serve with a side salad.

NUTRITION: Calories 161 Fat 5g Carbs 1g Protein 25g

Tender Lamb

Preparation time: 45 minutes
Cooking Time: 40 Minutes
Servings: 6

INGREDIENTS:
- 3 lamb shanks
- Seasoning mixture (1 tablespoon oregano, 1/4 teaspoon ground cumin and 1 tablespoon smoked paprika)
- 3 cloves garlic, minced
- 2 cups red wine
- 4 cups beef stock

DIRECTIONS:
1. Coat the lamb shanks with the seasoning mixture. Sprinkle with salt and pepper. Cover with minced garlic. Marinate in half of the mixture for 30 minutes. Set the Instant Pot to sauté. Pour in 2 tablespoons of olive oil. Brown the lamb on all sides. Remove and set aside. Add the rest of the ingredients.
2. Put the lamb back to the pot. Cover the pot and set it too manual. Cook at high pressure for 30 minutes. Release the pressure naturally. Set the

Instant Pot to sauté to simmer and thicken the sauce.

NUTRITION: Calories 566 Fat 29.4g Carbohydrate 12g Protein 48.7g

Worcestershire Pork Chops

Preparation time: 15 minutes
Cooking Time: 15 Minutes
Servings: 3

INGREDIENTS:

- ✓ 2 tablespoons Worcestershire sauce
- ✓ 8 oz pork loin chops
- ✓ 1 tablespoon lemon juice
- ✓ 1 teaspoon olive oil

DIRECTIONS:

1. Mix up together Worcestershire sauce, lemon juice, and olive oil. Brush the pork loin chops with the sauce mixture from each side. Preheat the grill to 395F.
2. Place the pork chops in the grill and cook them for 5 minutes. Then flip the pork chops on another side and brush with remaining sauce mixture. Grill the meat for 7-8 minutes more.

NUTRITION: Calories 267 Fat 20.4g Carbs 2.1g Protein 17g

Greek Pork

Preparation time: 15 minutes
Cooking Time: 50 Minutes
Servings: 8

INGREDIENTS:

- ✓ 3 lb. pork roast, sliced into cubes
- ✓ 1/4 cup chicken broth
- ✓ 1/4 cup lemon juice
- ✓ 2 teaspoons dried oregano
- ✓ 2 teaspoons garlic powder

DIRECTIONS:

1. Put the pork in the Instant Pot. In a bowl, mix all the remaining ingredients. Pour the mixture over the pork. Toss to coat evenly. Secure the pot.
2. Choose manual mode. Cook at high pressure for 50 minutes. Release the pressure naturally.

NUTRITION: Calories 478 Fat 21.6g Carbohydrate 1.2g Protein 65.1g

Pork with Green Beans & Potatoes

Preparation time: 15 minutes
Cooking Time: 22 Minutes
Servings: 6

INGREDIENTS:

- ✓ lb. lean pork, sliced into cubes
- ✓ 1 onion, chopped
- ✓ 2 carrots, sliced thinly
- ✓ 2 cups canned crushed tomatoes
- ✓ 2 potatoes, cubed

DIRECTIONS:

1. Set the Instant Pot to sauté. Add ½ cup of olive oil. Cook the pork for 5 minutes, stirring frequently. Add the rest of the ingredients. Mix well.
2. Seal the pot. Choose manual setting. Cook at high pressure for 17 minutes. Release the pressure naturally.

NUTRITION: Calories 428 Fat 24.4g Carbohydrate 27.6g Protein 26.7g

Beef and Chili Mix

Preparation time: 15 minutes

Cooking Time: 16 Minutes

Servings: 4

INGREDIENTS:

- ✓ 2 green chili peppers
- ✓ 8 oz beef flank steak
- ✓ 1 teaspoon salt
- ✓ 2 tablespoons olive oil
- ✓ 1 teaspoon apple cider vinegar

DIRECTIONS:

1. Pour olive oil in the skillet. Place the flank steak in the oil and roast it for 3 minutes from each side. Then sprinkle the meat with salt and apple cider vinegar.
2. Chop the chili peppers and add them in the skillet. Fry the beef for 10 minutes more. Stir it from time to time.

NUTRITION: Calories 166 Fat 10.5g Carbs 0.2g Protein 17.2g

Greek Meatballs

Preparation time: 15 minutes
Cooking Time: 10 Minutes
Servings: 8-10

INGREDIENTS:

- ✓ 2 lb. ground lamb
- ✓ 1 onion, chopped
- ✓ 1/4 cup fresh parsley, chopped
- ✓ 1/2 cup almond flour
- ✓ 1 teaspoon dried oregano

DIRECTIONS:

1. In a large bowl, combine all the ingredients. Mix well and form into small meatballs. Put the balls on the steamer basket inside the Instant Pot.
2. Pour in 1 cup of broth to the bottom of the pot. Secure the pot. Choose manual. Cook at high pressure for 10 minutes. Release the pressure quickly. While waiting, mix the rest of the ingredients.

NUTRITION: Calories 214 Fat 7.9g Carbohydrate 5.5g Protein 28.7g

Mediterranean Lamb Bowl

Preparation time: 15 minutes
Cooking time: 15 minutes
Servings: 2

INGREDIENTS:

- 2 tablespoons extra-virgin olive oil
- ¼ cup diced yellow onion
- 1 pound ground lamb
- 1 teaspoon dried mint
- 1 teaspoon dried parsley
- ½ teaspoon red pepper flakes
- ¼ teaspoon garlic powder
- 1 cup cooked rice
- ½ teaspoon za'atar seasoning
- ½ cup halved cherry tomatoes
- 1 cucumber, peeled and diced
- 1 cup store-bought hummus or Garlic-Lemon Hummus
- 1 cup crumbled feta cheese
- 2 pita breads, warmed (optional)

DIRECTIONS:

1. In a large sauté pan or skillet, heat the olive oil over medium heat and cook the onion for about 2 minutes, until fragrant.
2. Add the lamb and mix well, breaking up the meat as you cook. Once the lamb is halfway cooked, add mint, parsley, red pepper flakes, and garlic powder.
3. In a medium bowl, mix together the cooked rice and za'atar, then divide between individual serving bowls. Add the seasoned lamb, then top the bowls with the tomatoes, cucumber, hummus, feta, and pita (if using).

NUTRITION: Calories: 1,312 Protein: 62g Carbohydrates: 62g Fat: 96g

Lamb Burger

Preparation time: 15 minutes
Cooking time: 15 minutes
Servings: 4

INGREDIENTS:

- ✓ 1 pound ground lamb
- ✓ ½ small red onion, grated
- ✓ 1 tablespoon dried parsley
- ✓ 1 teaspoon dried oregano
- ✓ 1 teaspoon ground cumin
- ✓ 1 teaspoon garlic powder
- ✓ ½ teaspoon dried mint
- ✓ ¼ teaspoon paprika
- ✓ ¼ teaspoon kosher salt
- ✓ 1/8 teaspoon freshly ground black pepper
- ✓ Extra-virgin olive oil, for panfrying
- ✓ 4 pita breads, for serving (optional)
- ✓ Tzatziki Sauce, for serving (optional)
- ✓ Pickled Onions, for serving (optional)

DIRECTIONS:

1. In a bowl, combine the lamb, onion, parsley, oregano, cumin, garlic powder, mint, paprika, salt, and pepper. Divide the meat into 4 small balls and work into smooth discs.
2. In a large sauté pan or skillet, heat a drizzle of olive oil over medium heat or brush a grill with oil and set it too medium.
3. Cook the patties for 4 to 5 minutes on each side, until cooked through and juices run clear. Enjoy lamb burgers in pitas, topped with tzatziki sauce and pickled onions (if using).

NUTRITION: Calories: 328 Protein: 19g Carbohydrates: 2g Fat: 27g

Quick Herbed Lamb and Pasta

Preparation time: 15 minutes
Cooking time: 15 minutes
Servings: 4

INGREDIENTS:

- ✓ 3 thick lamb sausages, removed from casing and crumbled
- ✓ 1 medium shallot, chopped
- ✓ 1½ cups diced baby portobello mushrooms
- ✓ 1 teaspoon garlic powder
- ✓ 1 tablespoon extra-virgin olive oil
- ✓ 1 pound bean-based penne pasta
- ✓ 4 medium Roma tomatoes, chopped
- ✓ 1 (14.5-ounce) can crushed tomatoes
- ✓ 3 tablespoons heavy cream

DIRECTIONS:

1. Heat a large sauté pan or skillet over medium-high heat. Add the sausage to the skillet and cook for about 5 minutes, mixing and breaking the sausage up until the sausage is halfway cooked.

2. Reduce the heat to medium-low and add the shallot. Continue cooking for about 3 minutes, until they're soft.
3. Add the mushrooms, garlic powder, and olive oil and cook for 5 to 7 minutes, until the mushrooms have reduced in size by half and all the water is cooked out.
4. Meanwhile, bring a large pot of water to a boil and cook the pasta according to the package directions, until al dente. Drain and set aside.
5. To the skillet, add the chopped and canned tomatoes and cook for 7 to 10 minutes, until the liquid thickens slightly.
6. Reduce the heat and add the cream, mixing well. Plate the pasta first and top with the sausage mixture.

NUTRITION: Calories: 706 Protein: 45g Carbohydrates: 79g Fat: 31g

Marinated Lamb Kebabs with Crunchy Yogurt Dressing

Preparation time: 15 minutes
Cooking time: 15 minutes
Servings: 4

INGREDIENTS:

- ½ cup plain, unsweetened, full-fat Greek yogurt
- ¼ cup extra-virgin olive oil
- ¼ cup freshly squeezed lemon juice
- 1 teaspoon grated lemon zest
- 2 garlic cloves, minced
- 2 tablespoons honey
- 2 tablespoons balsamic vinegar
- 1½ teaspoons oregano, fresh, minced
- 1 teaspoon thyme, fresh, minced
- 1 bay leaf
- 1 teaspoon kosher salt
- ½ teaspoon freshly ground black pepper
- ½ teaspoon red pepper flakes
- 2 pounds leg of lamb, trimmed, cleaned and cut into 1-inch pieces

- ✓ 1 large red onion, diced large
- ✓ 1 recipe Crunchy Yogurt Dip
- ✓ Parsley, chopped, for garnish
- ✓ Lemon wedges, for garnish

DIRECTIONS:

1. In a bowl or large resealable bag, combine the yogurt, olive oil, lemon juice and zest, garlic, honey, balsamic vinegar, oregano, thyme, bay leaf, salt, pepper, and red pepper flakes. Mix well.
2. Add the lamb pieces and marinate, refrigerated, for 30 minutes. Preheat the oven to 375°F. Thread the lamb onto the skewers, alternating with chunks of red onion as desired.
3. Put the skewers onto a baking sheet and roast for 10 to 15 minutes, rotating every 5 minutes to ensure that they cook evenly.
4. Plate the skewers and allow them to rest briefly. Top or serve with the yogurt dressing. To finish, garnish with fresh chopped parsley and a lemon wedge.

NUTRITION: Calories: 578 Protein: 56g Carbohydrates: 20g Fat: 30g

Garlic Pork Tenderloin and Lemony Orzo

Preparation time: 15 minutes
Cooking time: 20 minutes
Servings: 6

INGREDIENTS:

- ✓ 1 pound pork tenderloin
- ✓ ½ teaspoon Shawarma Spice Rub
- ✓ 1 tablespoon salt
- ✓ ½ teaspoon coarsely ground black pepper
- ✓ ½ teaspoon garlic powder, 6 tablespoons extra-virgin olive oil
- ✓ 3 cups Lemony Orzo

DIRECTIONS:

- Preheat the oven to 350°F. Rub the pork with shawarma seasoning, salt, pepper, and garlic powder and drizzle with the olive oil.
- Put the pork on a baking sheet and roast for 20 minutes, or until desired doneness. Remove the pork from the oven and let rest for 10 minutes. Assemble the pork on a plate with the orzo and enjoy.

NUTRITION: Calories: 579 Protein: 33g Carbohydrates: 37g Fat: 34g

Roasted Pork with Apple-Dijon Sauce

Preparation time: 15 minutes
Cooking time: 40 minutes
Servings: 8

INGREDIENTS:

- ✓ 1½ tablespoons extra-virgin olive oil
- ✓ 1 (12-ounce) pork tenderloin
- ✓ ¼ teaspoon kosher salt
- ✓ ¼ teaspoon freshly ground black pepper
- ✓ ¼ cup apple jelly
- ✓ ¼ cup apple juice
- ✓ 2 to 3 tablespoons Dijon mustard
- ✓ ½ tablespoon cornstarch
- ✓ ½ tablespoon cream

DIRECTIONS:

1. Preheat the oven to 325°F. In a large sauté pan or skillet, heat the olive oil over medium heat.
2. Add the pork to the skillet, using tongs to turn and sear the pork on all sides. Once seared, sprinkle pork with salt and pepper, and set it on a small baking sheet.

3. In the same skillet, with the juices from the pork, mix the apple jelly, juice, and mustard into the pan juices. Heat thoroughly over low heat, stirring consistently for 5 minutes. Spoon over the pork.
4. Put the pork in the oven and roast for 15 to 17 minutes, or 20 minutes per pound. Every 10 to 15 minutes, baste the pork with the apple-mustard sauce.
5. Once the pork tenderloin is done, remove it from the oven and let it rest for 15 minutes. Then, cut it into 1-inch slices.
6. In a small pot, blend the cornstarch with cream. Heat over low heat. Add the pan juices into the pot, stirring for 2 minutes, until thickened. Serve the sauce over the pork.

NUTRITION: Calories: 146 Protein: 13g Carbohydrates: 8g Fat: 7g

Lightning Source UK Ltd.
Milton Keynes UK
UKHW021949140621
385519UK00002B/413